HEALTHY WEIGHT AFTER 40

Diet, Exercise, and Lifestyle Hacks for Healthy Weight Loss in Seniors.

Ann Bright

Table of contents

Introduction

Why Belly Fat After 40? A Battle Against Shifting Tides

The dreaded belly fat seems to appear with a vengeance around the age of 40, and can feel particularly stubborn to shed. This isn't just your imagination. There are several physiological changes happening around this time that can contribute to increased belly fat accumulation. Let's look into the key culprits:

Hormonal Shifts:

Estrogen (Women): For women, a major factor is the decline in estrogen levels that occurs during perimenopause and menopause. Estrogen helps regulate fat distribution, and with its decrease, fat tends to deposit more around the abdomen compared to the hips and thighs (the pre-menopausal pattern). This belly fat, particularly the visceral fat that sits deep within the abdomen, is linked to a higher risk of health problems like heart disease and type 2 diabetes.

Testosterone (Men): Men also experience hormonal changes, with a gradual decline in testosterone production starting around 30. Testosterone helps maintain muscle mass, and as levels drop, muscle mass can decrease. Muscle burns more calories than fat, so this decline can contribute to a slower metabolism and weight gain, often concentrated in the belly area.

Metabolic Slowdown:

Basal Metabolic Rate (BMR): Our BMR, the rate at which our body burns calories at rest, naturally slows down with age. This is partly due to the decrease in muscle mass mentioned earlier. A slower BMR means we need to consume fewer calories to maintain our weight, and any excess calories are more likely to be stored as fat.

Insulin Sensitivity: As we age, our bodies can become less sensitive to insulin, the hormone that regulates blood sugar. This can lead to increased blood sugar levels and a condition called insulin resistance. Insulin resistance can promote fat storage, particularly around the belly.

Other Lifestyle Factors:
Diet: Unhealthy eating habits, like consuming excessive sugar, processed foods, and unhealthy fats, can contribute to weight gain and belly fat accumulation.
Physical Activity: A decrease in physical activity levels is common with age. Regular exercise is crucial for maintaining muscle mass, boosting

metabolism, and promoting overall health. Lower activity levels can lead to weight gain, including belly fat.

Stress: Chronic stress can elevate cortisol levels, a stress hormone that can increase belly fat storage.

Taking Charge: Strategies to Reduce Belly Fat After 40

While these age-related changes can make belly fat more challenging to manage, it's definitely not a losing battle. Here are some strategies to combat belly fat and improve your health:

Diet: Focus on a balanced diet rich in whole foods like fruits, vegetables, whole grains, and lean protein. Limit processed foods, sugary drinks, and unhealthy fats.

Exercise: Aim for a combination of strength training to build muscle and cardio exercise to burn calories. Aim for at least 150 minutes of moderate-intensity exercise or 75 minutes of vigorous-intensity exercise per week. Strength training, 2-3 times a week, is also recommended.

Stress Management: Find healthy ways to manage stress, such as yoga, meditation, deep breathing exercises, or spending time in nature.

Quality Sleep: Aim for 7-8 hours of quality sleep each night. Poor sleep can disrupt hormones that regulate appetite and metabolism, making weight management more difficult.

Remember, consistency is key. By making sustainable changes to your diet and exercise routine, and managing stress, you can reduce belly fat, improve your overall health, and feel your best after 40. It's also important to consult your doctor before starting any new exercise program or making significant changes to your diet, especially if you have any underlying health conditions.

The Allure and Illusion of Spot Reduction: Why Targeted Exercises Won't Sculpt Your Dreams

The desire for a quick fix to target stubborn fat deposits is understandable. We've all seen the infomercials or social media posts promising sculpted abs or toned thighs with just a few minutes of targeted exercise. However, the concept of "spot reduction"—losing fat in a specific area through isolated exercises—is a persistent myth in the fitness world. Let's delve into the science behind why endless crunches won't magically flatten your belly, and explore more effective strategies for body composition goals.

Why Spot Reduction is a Myth:

Mobilization, Not Localization: Fat loss is a systemic process. When your body taps into stored fat for energy, it doesn't pull from specific areas. Exercise mobilizes fat stores from throughout the body, and genetics and hormones largely dictate where that fat will be released from first.

Muscle vs. Fat: Targeted exercises primarily build muscle, not burn fat directly. While building muscle can slightly boost your metabolism, it's not a magic bullet for spot reduction. Building muscle definition can however, give the illusion of a slimmer physique as muscle takes up less space than fat for the same weight.

The Flawed Logic of Targeted Exercises:

Let's dissect the logic behind common spot reduction exercises:

Crunches and Sit-Ups: While these exercises strengthen the abdominal muscles, they do little to burn significant belly fat. They target the superficial rectus abdominis muscle, not the deeper visceral fat that accumulates around the organs and is linked to health risks.

Spot Toning with Machines: Machines that isolate specific muscle groups might improve muscle tone, but again, won't directly target fat loss in that area.

Effective Strategies for Body Composition:

Here's what will help you achieve your body composition goals:

Focus on Overall Calorie Deficit: To lose weight and reduce fat stores, you need to create a calorie deficit – burning more calories than you consume. This can be achieved through a combination of healthy eating and exercise.

Embrace Compound Exercises: Compound exercises, like squats, lunges, push-ups, and rows, engage multiple muscle groups at once, burning more calories and promoting overall fitness.

Incorporate Cardio: Regular cardio exercise, such as brisk walking, running, swimming, or cycling, is crucial for burning calories and promoting overall fat loss. Aim for at least 150 minutes of moderate-intensity cardio or 75 minutes of vigorous-intensity cardio per week.

Strength Training for Overall Metabolism: Building muscle mass through strength training has a positive impact on your metabolism, even at rest. This means your body burns more calories throughout the day, even when you're not actively exercising.

Diet Plays a Crucial Role: A healthy diet rich in whole foods, fruits, vegetables, lean protein, and whole grains provides your body with the nutrients it needs and helps you feel full, reducing cravings and overeating. Limit processed foods, sugary drinks, and unhealthy fats.

Remember:

Focus on creating a sustainable lifestyle that incorporates healthy eating, regular exercise, and stress management. Consistency is key. Spot reduction might be a tempting myth, but by understanding the science of fat loss and implementing a holistic approach, you can achieve your body composition goals and improve your overall health.

Importance of Sustainable Change for Lasting weight Loss After 40

You've cracked open "Healthy weight After 40," and the promise of a trimmer waistline beckons. But before we dive into meal plans and exercise routines, let's address a crucial truth: **lasting weight loss hinges on sustainable change, not fleeting fads**. Crash diets and quick fixes might offer a temporary illusion of progress, but they're often unsustainable and ultimately lead to disappointment. This chapter is your roadmap to building healthy habits that will melt belly fat and empower you to keep it off for the long haul.

Why Quick Fixes Fail:

The allure of quick fixes is undeniable. We crave instant results, a magic bullet to erase stubborn belly fat. But these approaches often backfire for several reasons:

- **Unsustainable Practices**: Crash diets typically involve severe calorie restriction, elimination of entire food groups, or intense exercise regimens. These are difficult to maintain, leading to yo-yo dieting and rebound weight gain.
- **Nutrient Deficiencies:** Restrictive diets often lack essential nutrients, leading to fatigue, muscle loss, and a weakened immune system. Your body needs a balanced range of nutrients to function optimally and promote healthy metabolism.
- **Psychological Impact:** Quick fixes can foster a negative relationship with food and exercise. The constant struggle to restrict and deprive yourself can lead to feelings of guilt and shame.

The Power of Sustainable Change:

Instead of chasing fleeting trends, we need to build a foundation of healthy habits that fit seamlessly into our lives. **Here's why sustainable change is the key to melting belly fat after 40:**

Long-Term Success: Sustainable changes become a way of life, not a temporary inconvenience. You'll develop a healthy relationship with food and exercise, fostering long-term success and a sense of empowerment.
Focus on Wellness: It's not just about aesthetics; it's about feeling your best. Sustainable changes promote overall well-being, boosting your energy levels, mood, and overall health.
Flexibility for Life: Life happens. Unexpected events can disrupt your routine. Sustainable changes are adaptable. You can adjust portions, choose healthy alternatives when dining out, and find ways to stay active even with a busy schedule.

Building Your Sustainable Action Plan:

Now, let's translate this philosophy into actionable steps:

Start Small, Aim Big: Don't try to overhaul your life overnight. Begin with small, achievable goals, like adding a serving of vegetables to each meal or incorporating a brisk walk three times a week. Gradually build upon these successes.

Find Activities You Enjoy: Exercise shouldn't feel like punishment. Explore activities you genuinely enjoy, whether it's dancing, swimming, hiking, or joining a fitness class. Fun fuels motivation.

Make Smart Food Choices: Focus on whole, unprocessed foods. Prioritize fruits, vegetables, lean protein, and whole grains. Don't deprive yourself;

find healthy alternatives you love. **Portion control is key.**

Plan and Prep: Planning meals and snacks in advance reduces the temptation to grab unhealthy options when you're short on time. Meal prep can be a lifesaver on busy days.

Embrace Mindfulness: Develop a mindful approach to eating. Savor your food, chew thoroughly, and stop when you're comfortably full. Listen to your body's hunger cues.

Prioritize Sleep: Aim for 7-8 hours of quality sleep each night. Sleep deprivation disrupts hormones that regulate appetite and metabolism, hindering your fat-burning efforts.

Remember, Consistency is key. There will be days when motivation wanes. Don't beat yourself up if you miss a workout or indulge in a treat. Forgive yourself, get back on track, and celebrate your progress, no matter how small. Building sustainable change is a journey, not a destination. Embrace the process, and watch your belly fat melt away as you build a healthier, happier you.

This chapter is just the beginning. The following chapters will equip you with the tools you need to implement these strategies, with delicious recipes, practical exercise routines, and tips for overcoming common challenges. Let's work on achieving a healthy weight after 40 together for good!

Part 1:

Understanding Your Body After 40

Chapter 1:

The Science of Belly Fat - Understanding Your Enemy.

Belly fat pinches at our waistlines, digs into our clothes, and can leave us feeling self-conscious. But beyond aesthetics, belly fat, particularly visceral fat, poses a significant health threat. This chapter talks about the science of belly fat, differentiating between its types and unveiling the concerning health risks it can bring after 40.

The Two Faces of Belly Fat:

Not all belly fat are equal. Our bodies store fat in two main locations:

1. **Subcutaneous Fat**: This lies just beneath the skin, giving our bodies their shape and providing insulation. While excessive subcutaneous fat can contribute to weight gain, it's generally considered less harmful than the other type.

2. **Visceral Fat**: This deep belly fat, also known as visceral adipose tissue (VAT), lurks within the abdominal cavity, nestled around our organs like the liver, intestines, and pancreas. Visceral fat is metabolically active, releasing hormones and inflammatory chemicals that can wreak havoc on our health.

Why Visceral Fat is the Villain:

While both types of belly fat contribute to weight gain, visceral fat is the real villain of the story. Here's why:

Metabolic Disruption: Visceral fat releases free fatty acids and inflammatory markers into the bloodstream. These disrupt insulin sensitivity, a crucial hormone regulating blood sugar. This can lead to insulin resistance, a precursor to type 2 diabetes.

Chronic Inflammation: Visceral fat is a hotbed of inflammation, a chronic low-grade simmer that can damage blood vessels and contribute to a variety of health problems.

Increased Health Risks: Studies have linked excessive visceral fat to a heightened risk of the following:

- **Heart disease:** Visceral fat can increase bad (LDL) cholesterol and decrease good (HDL) cholesterol, promoting plaque buildup in arteries and raising the risk of heart attack and stroke.

- **Type 2 Diabetes:** As mentioned earlier, visceral fat disrupts insulin sensitivity, making it harder for your body to regulate blood sugar levels.

- **Certain Cancers:** Research suggests a link between visceral fat and an increased risk of some cancers, such as colon and pancreatic cancer.

- **Sleep Apnea:** Excess belly fat can put pressure on the diaphragm, making it harder to breathe during sleep, leading to sleep apnea.

- **Cognitive Decline:** Visceral fat may be linked to an increased risk of dementia and Alzheimer's disease.

The Age Factor:

As we enter our 40s, hormonal changes and a natural metabolic slowdown can make us more prone to accumulating visceral fat. Reduced estrogen levels in women and declining testosterone levels in men can contribute to a shift in fat storage patterns, favoring visceral fat deposition around the abdomen.

Identifying Your Risk:

While measuring your waist circumference isn't a foolproof method, it can be a good indicator of visceral fat. Here's a general guideline:

Men: A waist circumference exceeding 40 inches (102 cm) is considered high risk.

Women: A waist circumference exceeding 35 inches (88 cm) is considered high risk.

Taking Charge of Your Health:

Understanding the science of belly fat, particularly the risks associated with visceral fat, is the first step towards taking control of your health. The good news? You can significantly reduce your visceral fat content and mitigate these health risks through lifestyle changes. The following chapters will equip you with the tools you need to achieve lasting belly fat loss and a healthier you.

Chapter 2:

Hormonal Shifts and Metabolism - Navigating the Changing Tides After 40

As we approach our 40s, a subtle but significant shift occurs within. Our bodies, once governed by a youthful hormonal orchestra, begin to experience a change in melody. The hormones that once kept us feeling trim and energetic start to slow their tempo, impacting our metabolism and making weight management a more challenging endeavor. This chapter discusses about the hormonal changes that occur after 40, particularly focusing on estrogen and testosterone, and explores how they influence weight gain, specifically belly fat accumulation.

The Flunctuating Hormonal system:

Hormones in our bodies work together like a complex symphony. These chemical messengers, secreted by glands, play a crucial role in various bodily functions, including metabolism, appetite regulation, and fat storage. After 40, the rhythm of this hormonal orchestra starts to change, with some key instruments playing softer melodies. This disrupts the delicate balance that once kept our weight in check.

Estrogen's Fading Influence:

For women, a significant change occurs during perimenopause and menopause – the decline of estrogen production. Estrogen, once a champion of fat regulation, starts to sing a quieter tune.

Here's how this fading melody impacts weight management:

Fat Distribution: Estrogen helps regulate where fat is stored in the body. With declining levels, fat tends to redistribute, favoring visceral fat accumulation around the abdomen, as opposed to the subcutaneous fat deposited on the hips and thighs pre-menopause. This belly fat is metabolically more active and poses a greater health risk.

Satiety Signals: Estrogen also plays a role in regulating appetite. Decreased estrogen levels can lead to increased hunger and cravings, making it harder to maintain a healthy calorie intake. Women might find themselves feeling hungrier more often and struggling with portion control.

Testosterone's Waning Power:

Men also experience hormonal shifts, with testosterone production gradually declining after 30. While the impact might not be as dramatic as estrogen decline in women, testosterone plays a vital role in weight management:

Testosterone acts as a conductor for building and maintaining muscle mass. As levels decrease, muscle mass naturally starts to decline. Muscle burns more calories than fat at rest, so this decline contributes to a slower metabolism and can lead to weight gain, often concentrated around the midsection.

Fat Storage: Testosterone also influences where fat gets stored. Lower levels might lead to a shift towards increased belly fat accumulation, similar to the changes experienced by women with declining estrogen.

Beyond the Hormonal Symphony:

While hormonal changes are a significant factor in weight gain after 40, it's important to consider other contributing factors that can amplify the off-key notes in our internal orchestra:

Metabolic Slowdown: As we age, our basal metabolic rate (BMR) – the rate at which our bodies burn calories at rest – naturally slows down. This means we need to consume fewer calories to maintain our weight, adding another layer of complexity to weight management.

Lifestyle Habits: Decreased physical activity and changes in diet habits are common with age. We might find ourselves less motivated to exercise and more susceptible to unhealthy cravings. These lifestyle factors can exacerbate the weight gain associated with hormonal shifts.

Understanding the Dissonance:

By understanding how hormones like estrogen and testosterone influence weight management after 40, we can start to adapt our strategies and rewrite the dissonant parts of our hormonal symphony. The following chapters will explore practical solutions to counter the effects of hormonal changes, focusing on diet, exercise, and potential therapeutic options (always consult a doctor before considering any hormonal therapy). We'll learn how to create a new, healthier melody in our hormonal symphony, promoting weight management and overall well-being after 40.

Chapter 3:

The Mind-Body Connection - The Orchestra Beyond Biology in Weight Management.

We'velooked into the hormonal shifts and metabolic changes that can disrupt our weight management efforts after 40. However, the human body is a complex ecosystem, and weight management is influenced by more than just internal chemistry. This chapter explores the mind-body connection, focusing on the often-overlooked role of stress, sleep, and emotional health in managing weight. These factors act as powerful, yet unseen instruments in the orchestra of weight management, playing a vital role in the overall symphony of our health.

Stress: The Discordant Conductor

Chronic stress, a constant companion in today's world, can wreak havoc on our weight management symphony. When stressed, our bodies release cortisol, a hormone known as the "fight-or-flight" hormone. While cortisol has its purpose in the short term, chronically elevated levels can disrupt our weight management efforts in several ways:

Increased Cravings: Cortisol can trigger cravings for sugary, high-carb foods, as the body seeks a quick energy boost. These comfort foods often lead to unhealthy snacking and weight gain. Studies have shown a correlation between chronic stress and increased consumption of processed foods, sugary drinks, and unhealthy fats.

Disrupted Sleep Patterns: Chronic stress can make it difficult to fall asleep and stay asleep, leading to sleep deprivation. Sleep deprivation further disrupts hormones that regulate appetite and metabolism, making us hungrier and more likely to overeat. The stress response can also lead to restless sleep, hindering the restorative processes that occur during deep sleep. **Reduced Motivation for Exercise:** When stressed, we often neglect self-care activities like exercise. This lack of physical activity can lead to weight gain and a slower metabolism. The feeling of being overwhelmed by stress can make prioritizing exercise seem like an insurmountable task, creating a negative cycle.

Sleep: The Restorative Maestro

Sleep, often seen as a luxury, is a vital component of the weight management symphony. During sleep, our bodies release hormones that regulate appetite and metabolism. Here's how getting enough quality sleep can significantly aid in weight management:

Appetite Regulation: Sleep regulates hormones like **leptin** (promotes satiety) and **ghrelin** (stimulates hunger). Adequate sleep ensures these hormones are functioning optimally, helping us feel full and avoid overeating. Studies have shown a link between insufficient sleep and increased levels of ghrelin and decreased levels of leptin, promoting hunger and making it harder to control calorie intake.

Metabolic Boost: Deep sleep helps regulate insulin sensitivity, a key factor in blood sugar control. Proper sleep also promotes muscle growth and repair, which can boost metabolism. Deep sleep allows the body to repair itself and optimize metabolic processes, leading to more efficient calorie burning.

Improved Energy Levels: Adequate sleep improves energy levels throughout the day, making us more likely to engage in physical activity, further aiding in weight management. Feeling rested increases our motivation and ability to exercise effectively, creating a positive cycle for weight management.

Emotional Health: Setting the Tone

Our emotional well-being also plays a significant role in weight management. When we're struggling with negative emotions like anxiety or depression, we might resort to unhealthy coping mechanisms that can sabotage weight loss efforts:

Emotional Eating: Using food to numb difficult emotions can lead to overeating and unhealthy food choices. Emotional eating often involves reaching for quick, calorie-dense comfort foods that provide temporary relief but hinder long-term weight management goals.

Body Image: Negative body image and low self-esteem can make us less motivated to take care of ourselves through healthy eating and exercise. Feeling discouraged about our appearance can create a cycle of self-defeat, hindering our motivation to make positive lifestyle changes.

Harmonizing the Symphony

By understanding the mind-body connection, we can learn to manage stress, prioritize sleep, and cultivate emotional well-being, all of which contribute significantly to weight management. Here are some strategies to create a harmonious symphony in your weight management journey:

Stress Management Techniques: Explore stress-reduction techniques like:
- yoga,
- meditation,
- deep breathing exercises,
- spending time in nature,

- or listening to calming music.

Finding healthy ways to manage stress can help regulate cortisol levels and promote overall well-being.

Sleep Hygiene Practices: Develop good sleep hygiene practices, such as;

- establishing a regular sleep schedule,
- creating a relaxing bedtime routine, ensuring a sleep-conducive environment (dark, cool, and quiet),
- and avoiding stimulating activities like screen time before bed.

Prioritizing good sleep hygiene can significantly improve sleep quality and its positive effects on weight management.

Mindful Eating: Practice mindful eating, focusing on the taste, texture, and satiety cues of your food. Eat slowly and savor each bite. Mindful eating promotes a more conscious relationship with food, helps you avoid mindless overeating and makes you healthier.

Part 2:

Building a Sustainable Eating Plan.

Chapter 4:

Macronutrients for Success - Building the Foundation for Belly Fat Loss

We have explored the hormonal shifts, metabolic changes, and the mind-body connection that influence weight management after 40. Now, it's time to discuss the building blocks of a healthy diet – **macronutrients.** This chapter focuses on protein, healthy fats, and complex carbohydrates, explaining their importance and how they can play a crucial role in your belly fat loss journey.

The Macronutrient Trio:

Macronutrients, or macros for short, are the three main categories of nutrients our bodies need in relatively large amounts for energy, growth, and repair. Understanding the role of each macronutrient is essential for creating a healthy and sustainable diet that promotes belly fat loss:

Protein: The building blocks of life, protein plays a vital role in muscle building and repair, hormone regulation, and satiety (feeling full).

Healthy Fats: Contrary to popular belief, healthy fats are essential for our bodies. They provide sustained energy, support cell function, and aid in nutrient absorption.

Complex Carbohydrates: These slow-burning carbs provide sustained energy, promote gut health, and keep you feeling fuller for longer.

Protein: The Satiety Champion

Protein is a key player in our quest to melt belly fat. Here's why:

Increased Satiety: Protein is known for its satiating properties. It helps you feel full for longer, reducing cravings and preventing overeating, which can lead to weight gain and belly fat accumulation.

Muscle Building and Preservation: Muscle burns more calories than fat, even at rest. Building and maintaining muscle mass through adequate protein intake can boost your metabolism and aid in belly fat loss.

Thermogenic Effect: The body burns more calories digesting and utilizing protein compared to other macronutrients. This creates a slight thermogenic effect, further aiding in calorie burning.

Focus on Lean Protein Sources:

While protein is crucial, it's important to choose lean protein sources:

- ❖ Skinless chicken or turkey breast
- ❖ Fish and seafood
- ❖ Lean cuts of beef
- ❖ Eggs
- ❖ Beans and legumes
- ❖ Tofu and tempeh (vegetarian options)

Healthy Fats: Essential Partners, Not Enemies

Healthy fats are not the enemy when it comes to belly fat loss. In fact, they play a vital role which includes:

Satiety and Hormone Regulation: Healthy fats, like those found in avocados, nuts, and seeds, contribute to feeling full and satisfied. They also help regulate hormones that influence hunger and satiety.

Nutrient Absorption: Healthy fats aid in the absorption of essential vitamins like vitamins A, D, E, and K, which are crucial for overall health.

Inflammation Reduction: Healthy fats can help reduce inflammation, a chronic low-grade condition linked to visceral fat accumulation.

Embrace a Variety of Healthy Fats:

Here are some sources of healthy fats to include in your diet:

- ❖ Avocados
- ❖ Nuts and seeds (almonds, walnuts, chia seeds, flaxseeds)
- ❖ Olive oil
- ❖ Fatty fish (salmon, tuna).

Complex Carbohydrates: Fueling Your Body Wisely

Complex carbohydrates provide sustained energy and dietary fiber, both essential for belly fat loss:

Steady Energy Release: Complex carbs, unlike their refined counterparts, release glucose slowly into the bloodstream, preventing blood sugar spikes and crashes that can lead to cravings and overeating.

Fiber Powerhouse: Complex carbohydrates, like whole grains and vegetables, are rich in fiber. Fiber keeps you feeling full for longer, promotes gut health, and aids in digestion.

Choose Wisely and Focus on Whole Grains:

Here are some excellent sources of complex carbohydrates to prioritize:

- ❖ Whole grains (brown rice, quinoa, oats),
- ❖ Starchy vegetables (sweet potatoes, potatoes, corn),
- ❖ Fruits (berries, apples, pears),
- ❖ Legumes (beans, lentils).

The Macronutrient Balance:

The ideal balance of protein, healthy fats, and complex carbohydrates for you will depend on various factors like your age, activity level, and individual goals. However, a general starting point might be:

40% Protein: Promotes satiety and muscle building.

30% Healthy Fats: Supports cell function and nutrient absorption.

30% Complex Carbohydrates: Provides sustained energy and dietary fiber.

This is just a starting point, and consulting with a registered dietitian can help you create a personalized plan that aligns with your specific needs and preferences.

The Macronutrient Magic:

By incorporating a balanced approach to protein, healthy fats, and complex carbohydrates, you can create a foundation for a healthy diet that promotes belly fat loss after 40. Protein keeps you feeling.

Chapter 5:

Portion Control and Mindful Eating - Mastering the Art of Mindful Bites

We've explored the hormonal shifts, the mind-body connection, and the importance of macronutrients for belly fat loss. Now, it's time to delve into the practical aspects of eating – portion control and mindful eating. These strategies are crucial for managing hunger cues, preventing overeating, and ultimately, achieving your belly fat reduction goals.

The Portion Illusion:

In today's world of supersized portions, it's easy to lose track of how much we're actually consuming. This can lead to overeating, even with healthy foods. Here's why portion control matters:

Calorie Creep: Even small, seemingly insignificant portion increases can lead to a significant calorie surplus over time. This calorie creep can sabotage your weight loss efforts.

Satiety Signals: Our bodies take time to register satiety (feeling full). When we eat large portions quickly, we might miss these signals and end up overeating before feeling satisfied.

Mastering the Art of Portion Control:

Here are some strategies to master portion control and become a mindful eater:

Downsize Your Plates: Using smaller plates can create the illusion of a larger portion, helping you feel satisfied with a smaller amount of food.

Measure and Pre-Portion: Measure out your portions using measuring cups or spoons, especially for calorie-dense foods like nuts and seeds. Pre-portion snacks into individual containers to avoid mindless munching.

Mindful Eating Techniques: Practice mindful eating techniques like eating slowly, savoring each bite, and focusing on the taste, texture, and aroma of your food. This allows you to tune into your body's satiety cues and stop eating when you're comfortably full.

Read Food Labels: Pay attention to serving sizes on food labels. It's easy to underestimate how much you're actually consuming, particularly with processed foods.

Understanding Hunger Cues:

Hunger is a natural physiological response, but it's important to learn to differentiate true hunger from other cues:

Physical Hunger Cues: True hunger comes with physical sensations like an empty stomach, growling, or slight dizziness.

Emotional Hunger: We often confuse emotional cues like boredom, stress, or anxiety with hunger. Emotional eating can lead to overeating and unhealthy food choices.

Habitual Eating: Sometimes we eat out of habit, not because we're truly hungry. Mindful eating practices can help you become more aware of your hunger cues and avoid unnecessary snacking.

Strategies for Managing Hunger Cues:

Here are some ways to manage hunger cues and avoid overeating:

Stay Hydrated: Dehydration can sometimes mimic hunger pangs.

Drinking plenty of water throughout the day can help curb cravings and prevent unnecessary snacking.

Healthy Snacks: Having healthy snacks readily available can help satisfy hunger pangs between meals. Choose options like fruits, vegetables, nuts, or yogurt.

Plan Your Meals: Planning your meals and snacks in advance can help you avoid unhealthy choices when hunger strikes.

Mindful Eating: Cultivating a Sustainable Approach.

Mindful eating is not just about portion control; it's about cultivating a healthy and sustainable relationship with food. Here are some benefits of mindful eating:

Reduced Stressful Eating: Mindful eating can help you identify emotional triggers for overeating and develop healthier coping mechanisms.

Appreciation for Food: Mindful eating allows you to savor the taste, texture, and aroma of your food, creating a more enjoyable eating experience.

Improved Dietary Choices: Paying closer attention to how your body reacts to different foods can help you make informed dietary choices that promote overall well-being.

The Power of Mindful Bites:

By mastering portion control and practicing mindful eating, you can empower yourself to make conscious choices about what and how much you eat. This approach can be a powerful tool in managing hunger cues, preventing overeating, and ultimately, achieving your belly fat loss goals. The next chapter will delve into creating a personalized exercise plan to complement your dietary efforts, creating a well-rounded approach for successful belly fat reduction.

Chapter 6:

Power Up with Anti-Inflammatory Foods - Fueling Your Fight Against Belly Fat

We have explored the hormonal changes, the mind-body connection, the importance of macronutrients, and strategies for mindful eating. Now, it's time to delve deeper into the world of food and its powerful role in belly fat reduction. This chapter focuses on anti-inflammatory foods, highlighting the importance of fruits, vegetables, whole grains, and healthy fats in your fight against belly fat and promoting overall well-being.

The Inflammation Connection:

Chronic low-grade inflammation is increasingly recognized as a contributing factor to various health issues, including obesity and weight gain, particularly belly fat accumulation. Certain foods can trigger inflammatory responses in the body, while others possess potent anti-inflammatory properties. By incorporating an anti-inflammatory diet rich in specific fruits, vegetables, whole grains, and healthy fats, you can empower your body to fight back against inflammation and support your belly fat loss journey.

The Powerhouse of Produce:

Fruits and vegetables are the cornerstone of an anti-inflammatory diet. They are packed with essential vitamins, minerals, antioxidants, and fiber, all of which play a role in reducing inflammation.

Antioxidant Power: Fruits and vegetables are rich in antioxidants, which combat free radicals that contribute to inflammation.

Fiber for a Healthy Gut: Dietary fiber, abundant in fruits and vegetables, promotes a healthy gut microbiome. A balanced gut microbiome is linked to reduced inflammation throughout the body.

Nutrient Richness: The vitamins and minerals found in fruits and vegetables are essential for various bodily functions, including regulating hormones and metabolism, which can indirectly influence inflammation.

Embrace a Rainbow on Your Plate:

Aim for a variety of colorful fruits and vegetables to reap the benefits of a wide range of antioxidants and other protective nutrients

Fruits: Berries (blueberries, strawberries, raspberries), citrus fruits (oranges, grapefruits), apples, pears, kiwifruit.

Vegetables: Leafy greens (spinach, kale), cruciferous vegetables (broccoli, cauliflower), bell peppers, sweet potatoes, carrots, tomatoes

Whole Grains: Fueling Your Body with Goodness

Whole grains provide sustained energy, keep you feeling full, and offer anti-inflammatory benefits which includes:

Fiber Power: Whole grains are a rich source of fiber, which promotes gut health and reduces inflammation.

Nutrient Package: Whole grains offer essential vitamins, minerals, and antioxidants that contribute to overall well-being.

Blood Sugar Regulation: Whole grains release glucose slowly into the bloodstream, helping to prevent blood sugar spikes and crashes that can trigger inflammatory responses.

Incorporate a Variety of Whole Grains

Here are some excellent whole-grain options to include in your diet:

- ❖ Brown rice,
- ❖ Quinoa,
- ❖ Oats,
- ❖ Whole-wheat bread and pasta,
- ❖ Barley.

Healthy Fats: Your Body's Anti-Inflammatory Allies.

Don't be afraid of healthy fats! They play a crucial role in reducing inflammation and offer a multitude of health benefits:

Anti-Inflammatory Properties: Certain healthy fats, like those found in fatty fish and olive oil, possess anti-inflammatory properties that can help combat belly fat accumulation.

Satiety and Hormone Regulation: Healthy fats promote satiety and aid in hormone regulation, both of which can contribute to weight management.

Nutrient Absorption: Healthy fats aid in the absorption of essential vitamins like vitamins A, D, E, and K, which are crucial for overall health and can indirectly influence inflammation.

Choose Wisely and Focus on Quality Fats:

Here are some excellent sources of healthy fats to incorporate into your anti-inflammatory diet:

- Fatty fish (salmon, tuna, sardines),
- Avocados,

- Nuts and seeds (almonds, walnuts, flaxseeds, chia seeds),
- Olive oil.

Building Your Anti-Inflammatory Plate:

By focusing on fruits, vegetables, whole grains, and healthy fats, you can create a powerful anti-inflammatory diet that supports your belly fat reduction efforts. Here are some tips for building your anti-inflammatory plate:

Fill half your plate with non-starchy vegetables: This ensures a good intake of fiber and essential nutrients.

Include a quarter plate of whole grains: It provides sustained energy and keeps you feeling full.

Add a serving of lean protein: which promotes satiety and muscle building.

Don't forget the healthy fats: Include a source of healthy fats like avocado or nuts to enhance satiety and nutrient absorption.

The Anti-Inflammatory Advantage:

An anti-inflammatory diet offers numerous benefits beyond belly fat reduction which includes:

- **Improved Overall Health:** Reducing inflammation can support overall well-being and potentially reduce the risk of chronic diseases.
- Enhanced Energy.

Chapter 7:

Taming Sugar Cravings - Conquering Your Sweet Tooth for Lasting Results

The battle against belly fat often feels like a war against sugar cravings. Those intense desires for sugary treats can derail even the most well-intentioned weight loss efforts. This chapter delves into the science behind sugar cravings, explores strategies for reducing your sugar intake, and introduces healthy alternatives to satisfy your sweet tooth, all to empower you on your journey to lasting results.

The Allure of Sugar:

Sugar, particularly refined sugar and high-fructose corn syrup, is a ubiquitous ingredient in our modern diet. Here's why it can be so addictive:

Blood Sugar Rollercoaster: Sugar causes rapid spikes in blood sugar, followed by sharp crashes. These crashes trigger cravings for more sugar to restore blood sugar levels, creating a vicious cycle.

Dopamine Reward: Sugar activates the reward center in the brain, releasing dopamine, a neurotransmitter associated with pleasure and motivation. This reinforces the desire for sugary foods.

Hidden Sugars: Many processed foods contain surprisingly high amounts of added sugar, making it easy to consume more than you realize.

Breaking the Sugar Chains:

While sugar cravings can be intense, there are strategies to reduce your reliance on sugary treats.

1. **Gradual Reduction:** Avoid the temptation to stop abruptly. Gradually reduce your sugar intake over time to allow your taste buds to adjust and to minimize withdrawal symptoms.
2. Identify Your Triggers: Pay attention to situations that trigger sugar cravings. Are you stressed, bored, or tired? Develop healthy coping mechanisms to address these triggers, such as exercise, meditation, or drinking a glass of water.
3. **Focus on Whole Foods**: Prioritize whole, unprocessed foods like fruits, vegetables, and whole grains. These foods naturally contain sugars but also provide fiber, vitamins, and minerals that help regulate blood sugar and promote satiety.
4. Read Food Labels: Learn how to read labels. Be mindful of added sugars lurking in seemingly

healthy products like yogurt, salad dressings, and granola bars.

Healthy Alternatives to Satisfy Your Sweet Tooth:

There's good news! You can satisfy your sweet tooth without succumbing to sugary treats. Here are some healthy alternatives:

Fruits: Nature's candy! Fruits provide sweetness along with fiber, vitamins, and minerals. Enjoy a piece of fruit with a dollop of nut butter for added protein and healthy fats.

Dates and Dried Fruits: Dates offer natural sweetness and a chewy texture. Use them in moderation, as they are calorie-dense. Unsweetened dried fruits can also be a satisfying option.

Dark Chocolate: Dark chocolate (70% cacao or higher) offers antioxidants and a satisfying dose of chocolate flavor.

Enjoy a small square to curb your cravings.

Sweetened with Spices: Experiment with spices like cinnamon, nutmeg, and ginger to add sweetness to yogurt, oatmeal, or baked goods.

Homemade Treats: Control the ingredients by making your own healthy desserts using natural sweeteners like honey, maple syrup, or dates.

Beyond Sugar Substitutes:

While sugar substitutes might seem like a quick fix, they're not a magic bullet. Here's why:

Not a Free Pass: Sugar substitutes can still trigger cravings and may disrupt your gut microbiome.

Focus on Long-Term Solutions: The goal is to develop a healthy relationship with food, not rely on artificial substitutes.

Taming the Cravings:

By employing these strategies, you can gradually tame your sugar cravings and break free from their hold.

Remember:

Be Patient: Changing habits takes time. Be patient with yourself and celebrate your progress.
Find Healthy Pleasures: Discover healthy ways to indulge your taste buds. Experiment with new recipes and healthy flavor combinations.
Focus on Overall Well-being: View your dietary changes as a journey towards a healthier, happier you. This shift in perspective can be a powerful motivator.

The Sweet Reward of Success:

By conquering your sugar cravings, you'll not only be on your way to achieving your belly fat loss goals, but you'll also be setting yourself up for a lifetime of healthy eating habits. The next chapter will delve into the world of exercise, exploring its role in belly fat reduction and providing guidance on creating a safe and effective exercise routine.

Part 3:

Exercise for a Stronger, Leaner You

Chapter 8:

Move Your Body: The Importance of Exercise for Lasting Success

We've explored the hormonal shifts, the mind-body connection, the importance of macronutrients, mindful eating strategies, and taming sugar cravings. Now, it's time to look into the importance of movement – **exercise.** This chapter explores the multifaceted benefits of exercise for weight management and overall health, empowering you to integrate physical activity into your belly fat reduction journey for lasting success.

Exercise: The Missing Piece of the Puzzle

While diet plays a crucial role in weight management, exercise is the missing piece of the puzzle for sustainable belly fat loss and overall well-being. Here's why:

Calorie Burning: Exercise burns calories, creating a calorie deficit that promotes weight loss. The intensity and duration of your workout determine the number of calories burned.

Muscle Building and Preservation: Muscle burns more calories than fat, even at rest. Building and maintaining muscle mass through exercise can boost your metabolism and aid in belly fat reduction.

Increased Insulin Sensitivity: Exercise improves your body's ability to utilize insulin, a hormone that regulates blood sugar levels. This helps prevent blood sugar spikes and crashes that can lead to cravings and overeating.

Exercise Benefits Beyond Weight Management:

The benefits of exercise extend far beyond weight management. Other benefits include:

- **Improved Cardiovascular Health:** Regular exercise strengthens your heart, improves blood circulation, and lowers your risk of heart disease, stroke, and high blood pressure.
- **Enhanced Mood and Reduced Stress:** Exercise releases endorphins, hormones that have mood-boosting and stress-reducing effects. Physical activity can be a powerful tool for managing stress and anxiety.
- **Stronger Bones and Joints:** Exercise strengthens bones and muscles, improving balance and coordination. This can help

prevent falls and injuries, especially as we age.

- **Improved Sleep Quality:** Regular physical activity can promote better sleep quality, providing you with the energy you need to tackle your day and manage your weight loss efforts effectively.

Finding Your Exercise Fit:

The key to successful exercise is finding activities you enjoy and can incorporate into your lifestyle. Here are some tips to get you started:

1. **Start Slowly:** If you're new to exercise, begin with low-impact activities like walking or swimming and gradually increase intensity and duration as your fitness level improves.
2. **Explore Different Activities:** Find activities you enjoy. This

could be dancing, biking, yoga, swimming, team sports, or even gardening.

3. **Make it a Habit:** Aim for at least 150 minutes of moderate-intensity exercise or 75 minutes of vigorous-intensity exercise per week. Break it down into manageable chunks throughout the day, like taking a brisk walk during your lunch break.

4. **Find a Workout Buddy:** Enlist a friend or family member to join you for your workouts. Having an exercise partner can increase accountability and make workouts more enjoyable.

Listen to Your Body:

It's important to listen to your body when exercising.

Warm-up and Cool-down: Always warm up before your workout to prepare your muscles and cool down afterward to promote recovery.

Rest and Recovery: Schedule rest days to allow your body to recover and prevent injuries.

Pay Attention to Pain: If you experience pain, stop the activity and consult a healthcare professional.

Exercise: Your Investment in a Healthier You

Exercise is an investment in your present and future health. By incorporating physical activity into your routine, you'll not only be on your way to achieving your belly fat loss goals, but you'll also be reaping a multitude of benefits for your overall well-being. The next chapter will provide a sample exercise plan to get you started and offer guidance on tailoring it to your individual needs and preferences. Remember, consistency is key! The more you move your body, the more

you'll reap the rewards of an active
lifestyle.

Chapter 9:

Strength Training: Building Muscle After 40 - Igniting Your Metabolism and Shaping Your Success

We have explored the hormonal changes, the mind-body connection, the importance of macronutrients, mindful eating strategies, taming sugar cravings, and the significance of exercise in weight management. Now, we will look deeper into the world of exercise, focusing on strength training. This chapter explores the benefits of strength training specifically for those over 40, highlighting its impact on metabolism and body composition, ultimately empowering you to shape your success in fat reduction.

Strength Training: Beyond Looking Good, Feeling Great.

Strength training, often associated with building bulky muscles, offers a multitude of benefits that extend far beyond aesthetics. Here's why strength training is a crucial component of your fat reduction plan, especially after 40:

Metabolic Boost: Muscle is metabolically active tissue. Building and maintaining muscle mass through strength training can increase your resting metabolic rate (RMR), the number of calories your body burns at rest. This translates to burning more calories throughout the day, even when you're not exercising.

Combating Age-Related Muscle Loss: As we age, we naturally experience muscle loss, a condition known as sarcopenia. Strength training helps combat this process, preserving muscle mass and its metabolic benefits.

Improved Body Composition: Strength training not only builds muscle but can also help reduce body fat percentage. This shift in body composition, with more muscle and less fat, leads to a leaner and more sculpted physique.

Stronger Bones and Joints: Strength training strengthens bones and improves joint stability, reducing the risk of osteoporosis and injuries, especially important as we age.

Enhanced Functional Fitness: Everyday activities become easier with increased strength. Carrying groceries, climbing stairs, and even gardening become less taxing.

Strength Training for Everyone:

Strength training is beneficial for people of all ages and fitness levels. Here are some tips to get you started on your strength training journey after 40:

1. **Start with Bodyweight Exercises:** Bodyweight exercises like squats, lunges, push-ups, and planks are a great way to begin building strength without any equipment.
2. **Consider Resistance Bands:**Resistance bands offer a safe and affordable way to add variety and intensity to your workouts.
3. **Free Weights or Weight Machines**: As you progress, consider incorporating free weights or weight machines into your routine. Always consult a certified personal trainer to learn proper form and technique to prevent injuries.
4. **Focus on Compound Exercises:** Compound exercises work multiple muscle groups

simultaneously, maximizing your workout efficiency. Examples include squats, deadlifts, rows, and presses.

5. **Listen to Your Body:** Start with lighter weights and gradually increase intensity as you get stronger. Pay attention to proper form and don't hesitate to ask a trainer for guidance.

Samples of Strength Training Routine:

Here are samples of beginner-friendly strength training routine to get you started. Perform each exercise for 10-12 repetitions, completing 2-3 sets per exercise. Rest for 30-60 seconds between sets.

Warm-up: 5-10 minutes of light cardio (brisk walking, jumping jacks) and dynamic stretches.

Squats: Targets your quads, glutes, and hamstrings.

Lunges: Works your legs and core for balance.

Push-ups (modified on knees if needed): Strengthens your chest, shoulders, and triceps.

Rows (using bodyweight, resistance bands, or weights): Works your back muscles and biceps.

Plank: Engages your core muscles for stability.

Cool-down: 5-10 minutes of static stretches to improve flexibility and prevent muscle soreness.

Remember, consistency is key! Aim for strength training sessions 2-3 times per week, allowing rest days for muscle recovery.

Strength training is an investment in your health and well-being, especially after 40. By incorporating strength training into your routine, you'll be:

- Boosting your metabolism and burning more calories.
- Building muscle and improving body composition.
- Strengthening your bones and joints.
- Enhancing your functional fitness and overall well-being.

The combined benefits of strength training and a healthy diet will empower you to achieve your fat reduction goals and shape your success for a healthier, stronger you.

Chapter 10:

High-Intensity Interval Training (HIIT) for Fat Burning - Unleashing the Afterburner Effect.

We have discussed about the hormonal changes, the mind-body connection, the importance of macronutrients, mindful eating strategies, taming sugar cravings, the significance of exercise in weight management, and the benefits of strength training. Here, we will discuss specific exercise modalities – specifically High-Intensity Interval Training (HIIT). This chapter explores the science behind HIIT, highlighting its effectiveness for boosting metabolism and aiding in fat burning, particularly for belly fat reduction.

HIIT is a training style characterized by alternating periods of intense anaerobic exercise with brief recovery periods. This creates a demanding yet efficient workout that can be a powerful tool for fat loss. Here's what makes HIIT so effective:

1. **The Afterburner Effect:** HIIT elevates your metabolic rate (the number of calories you burn) not just during the workout but also for hours afterward. This "afterburner effect" helps you burn more calories at rest, promoting fat loss.

2. **Increased Fitness Level:** HIIT improves your cardiovascular health and VO2 max (the maximum amount of oxygen your body can utilize during exercise). This overall fitness boost contributes to a higher basal metabolic rate, leading to more calorie burning throughout the day.

3. **Muscle Preservation:** Unlike traditional cardio, which can lead to muscle loss, HIIT can help preserve muscle mass, further enhancing your metabolism. Muscle burns more calories than fat, even at rest.

While HIIT workouts can be intense, they are adaptable to various fitness levels:

Beginner Modifications: Beginners can start with shorter intervals, lower intensity levels, and longer recovery periods. Modify exercises to suit your fitness level.

Scalability: As your fitness improves, you can gradually increase the intensity, duration of intervals, and decrease rest periods for a more challenging workout.

Sample HIIT Routine:

Here's a sample beginner-friendly HIIT routine to get you started. Perform each exercise for 30 seconds at high intensity, followed by 60 seconds of rest. Repeat the entire circuit 2-3 times.

Jumping Jacks: A classic cardio exercise that gets your heart rate up.
Squats: Targets your quads, glutes, and hamstrings.
High Knees: A running motion in place, good for cardio and core engagement.
Mountain Climbers: A dynamic exercise that works your core, legs, and arms.
Rest: Take a full 60 seconds of rest to allow your heart rate to recover before the next round.

Remember, listen to your body! If you experience any pain, stop the workout and consult a healthcare professional.

HIIT is a time-efficient and effective way to boost your metabolism, burn calories, and promote belly fat reduction. Here are some additional benefits of incorporating HIIT into your routine:

- **Improved Overall Fitness**: HIIT enhances cardiovascular health, improves VO2 max, and strengthens muscles.
- **Increased Energy Levels**: Regular HIIT workouts can boost your energy levels and leave you feeling more energized throughout the day.
- **Time-Efficient**: HIIT workouts can be completed in a shorter time compared to traditional cardio sessions, making them ideal for busy schedules.

Remember, consistency is key to achieving your fitness goals. Aim for 2-3 HIIT workouts per week, allowing rest days for recovery. Combine HIIT with a healthy diet and strength training for a well-rounded belly fat reduction strategy. With dedication and the right tools, you can achieve lasting results and feel your best.

Disclaimer: As with any exercise program, consult with your healthcare professional before starting HIIT, especially if you have any pre-existing health conditions. They can help you determine if HIIT is safe and appropriate for you and can guide you on proper form and technique to prevent injuries.

Chapter 11:

Finding Activities You Love - Making Exercise a Joyful Journey

Now, we arrive at a crucial chapter: finding activities you love. This might seem counterintuitive – exercise is often viewed as a chore, not a source of enjoyment. But here's the secret: when you discover activities you genuinely enjoy, exercise transforms from a burden into a joyful journey that fuels your fat reduction efforts and overall well-being.

The Power of Enjoyment:

Here's why prioritizing activities you enjoy is crucial for sustainable exercise:

Increased Motivation: When you look forward to your workouts, you're more likely to stick with them in the long run.

Reduced Stress: Exercise should feel like a stress reliever, not a stressor. Choosing activities you enjoy promotes relaxation and enjoyment.

Improved Consistency: When exercise feels like a chore, skipping workouts becomes easier. Finding activities you love makes consistency more natural.

Enhanced Mood: Physical activity releases endorphins, the body's natural feel-good chemicals. Choosing activities you enjoy intensifies this mood-boosting effect.

Unleashing Your Inner Athlete:

So, how do you find activities you love? Here are some strategies to explore:

- **Reflect on Past Enjoyments:** Did you enjoy team sports in your younger years? Or maybe you loved dancing? Reconnect with activities that brought you joy in the past.

- **Explore New Options**: Step outside your comfort zone! Try a Zumba class, a rock climbing session, or a kayaking adventure. You might discover a hidden passion.

- **Embrace the Outdoors:** Nature provides a beautiful backdrop for exercise. Take a hike, go for a bike ride, or try stand-up paddleboarding.

- **Find a Workout Buddy**: Enlist a friend or family member to join you for your workouts. Shared experiences can make exercise more fun and motivating.

- **Embrace Technology**: Explore fitness apps or online workout videos that offer a variety of activities and routines. You might find a virtual class you love.

- **Listen to Your Body (and Your Heart):**

Finding activities you love is a journey of exploration:

- **Be Open-Minded:** Not every activity will be a perfect fit. Try different things and be open to discovering new passions.
- **Don't Be Afraid to Quit:** If you truly dislike an activity, don't force yourself to do it. There are countless other options waiting to be explored.
- **Focus on Progress, Not Perfection**: Celebrate your progress, no matter how small. Each workout is a step in the right direction.

Making Exercise a Habit:

Here are some tips to transform your newfound love for exercise into a sustainable habit:

Schedule Your Workouts: Treat your exercise sessions like important appointments. Block out time in your calendar and stick to it.

Start Small and Gradually Increase: Don't overwhelm yourself. Begin with shorter workouts and gradually increase duration and intensity as your fitness level improves.

Reward Yourself: Celebrate your achievements! After reaching a fitness goal, reward yourself with something non-food related, like a massage or a new workout outfit.

Find a Support System: Surround yourself with positive and supportive people who encourage your healthy lifestyle choices.

Exercise as Lifelong Journey, Not a Short-Term Fix:

Finding activities you love is about making exercise a lifelong journey, not a short-term fix for belly fat reduction. When you prioritize enjoyment, exercise becomes a source of physical and mental well-being, contributing to a healthier and happier you. Here are some additional benefits of prioritizing activities you love:

Increased Confidence: Regular exercise can improve your body image and boost your overall confidence.

Stress Management: Physical activity is a potent tool for managing stress and anxiety.

Better Sleep: Regular exercise promotes better quality sleep, leaving you feeling more energized throughout the day.

Improved Overall Health: Exercise reduces your risk of chronic diseases like heart disease, diabetes, and certain types of cancer.

The Final Takeaway:

Exercise doesn't have to be a chore. By prioritizing activities you enjoy and making movement a joyful experience, you'll be well on your way to achieving your belly fat reduction goals and creating a foundation for a lifetime of health and well-being. Remember, the most important step is to begin. So, lace up your shoes, put on your favorite music, and step out the door. You might just surprise yourself with how much you enjoy the journey!

Part 4:

Lifestyle Habits for Long-Term Success.

Chapter 12:

The Power of Sleep: Unlocking Your Body's Natural Fat-Burning Potential.

In our quest for lasting fat reduction, we've explored various strategies – understanding hormonal influences, crafting a balanced diet, incorporating exercise routines we enjoy. Now, let's delve into a powerful yet often overlooked factor: **sleep**. This chapter looks deep into the science behind sleep, revealing its profound impact on weight management and overall health. You'll discover how prioritizing quality sleep unlocks your body's natural fat-burning potential and empowers you on your journey towards a healthier, happier you.

Sleep: Beyond Resting Your Eyes

While sleep may seem like a passive state of shutting down, it's actually a period of intense biological activity. During sleep, your body orchestrates a symphony of essential tasks: repairing tissues, consolidating memories, and regulating hormones that play a crucial role in weight management and overall health. Here's why prioritizing quality sleep is a fundamental pillar for fat reduction:

Hormonal Harmony: Sleep acts as a conductor for hormones like leptin (the satiety hormone) and ghrelin (the hunger hormone). When sleep is inadequate, this delicate balance gets disrupted. Leptin production decreases, leading to decreased feelings of fullness, while ghrelin production increases, fueling hunger pangs and cravings for high-calorie foods. This hormonal imbalance can significantly hinder your weight management efforts.

Metabolic Boost: Sleep deprivation can negatively impact your metabolism, the process by which your body converts food into energy. When sleep-deprived, your body becomes less efficient at burning calories, making it harder to lose weight and maintain a healthy energy level.

Insulin Sensitivity: Sleep plays a vital role in regulating insulin, a hormone that helps your body absorb glucose (sugar) from the bloodstream. Chronic sleep deprivation can lead to insulin resistance, a condition where your cells become less responsive to insulin. This can contribute to weight gain and increase your risk of developing type 2 diabetes.

Appetite Control: Sleep deprivation disrupts the communication between your brain and stomach. When sleep-deprived, your brain may not receive the signals indicating satiety, leading to overeating and unhealthy food choices.

The Ripple Effect of Sleep Deprivation:

The consequences of chronic sleep deprivation extend far beyond hindering weight management. They includes:

Decreased Immunity: Sleep is essential for a healthy immune system. When sleep-deprived, your body produces fewer infection-fighting cells, making you more susceptible to illness.

Cognitive Decline: Sleep is crucial for memory consolidation and learning. Sleep deprivation can impair cognitive function, focus, and decision-making abilities.

Mood Swings: Sleep deprivation can exacerbate mood swings, anxiety, and depression. You might experience increased frustration, irritability, and difficulty managing stress.

Increased Risk of Chronic Diseases: Chronic sleep deprivation is linked to an increased risk of chronic diseases like heart disease, stroke, and type 2 diabetes.

How Much Sleep Do You Need?

The National Sleep Foundation recommends that adults get between 7 and 9 hours of sleep per night. However, individual needs may vary. Listen to your body and aim for the amount of sleep that leaves you feeling refreshed, energized, and focused throughout the day.

Creating a Sleep Sanctuary:

Here are some practical tips to create a sleep-conducive environment and promote better sleep hygiene:

- **Establish a Regular Sleep Schedule**: Go to bed and wake up at consistent times, even on weekends. This helps regulate your body's natural sleep-wake cycle, known as your circadian rhythm. Consistency allows your body to anticipate sleep and wakefulness, promoting easier falling asleep and waking up feeling refreshed.

- **Develop a Relaxing Bedtime Routine**: Wind down before bed with calming activities that signal to your body it's time to prepare for sleep. This could include taking a warm bath, reading a book, practicing deep breathing or meditation techniques, or listening to calming music. Avoid activities that stimulate the brain, such as watching television or working on electronic devices.

- **Optimize Your Sleep Environment**: Make sure your

bedroom is a haven for sleep. It should be dark, quiet, cool, and clutter-free. Invest in blackout curtains or an eye mask to block out light. Use earplugs or a white noise machine to minimize noise disruptions. Ensure your bedroom temperature is cool, ideally between 60-67 degrees Fahrenheit.

- **Limit Screen Time Before Bed**: The blue light emitted from electronic devices like smartphones, laptops, and tablets can disrupt sleep patterns by suppressing melatonin production, a hormone that regulates your sleep-wake cycle. Avoid screen time for at least an hour before bedtime.
- **Regular Exercise**: Regular physical activity can improve sleep quality. However, avoid strenuous workouts close to bedtime, as they can have a stimulating effect.

- **Manage Stress**: Chronic stress can significantly impact sleep.

Chapter 13:

Managing Stress and Finding Calm - Cultivating Inner Peace for Weight Management Success.

Now, let's talk about a crucial factor that can significantly impact all the already discussed aspects: **stress**. This chapter explores the link between stress and weight management, and equips you with powerful techniques for stress reduction and relaxation. By cultivating inner peace, you'll not only feel better overall, but also empower your weight management efforts.

Stress: The Silent Saboteur

Stress is a natural human response to challenging situations. However, chronic stress can wreak havoc on your body and mind, hindering your weight management goals. Here's how:

Cortisol Chaos: When stressed, your body releases cortisol, a hormone that promotes the storage of belly fat. Chronic stress keeps cortisol levels elevated, leading to increased belly fat accumulation.

Craving Control: Stress can trigger unhealthy coping mechanisms like emotional eating. You might find yourself reaching for sugary or high-fat foods for comfort, leading to weight gain.

Sleepless Nights: Stress can disrupt your sleep patterns, making it harder to fall asleep and stay asleep. As discussed in the previous chapter, sleep deprivation can disrupt hormones, decrease metabolism, and increase cravings, further hindering weight management.

The Benefits of Stress Management:

Learning effective stress management techniques offers numerous benefits beyond weight control:

- **Improved Overall Health**: Chronic stress weakens your immune system, making you more susceptible to illness. Stress management techniques can improve your physical health and well-being.
- **Enhanced Mood**: Chronic stress can contribute to anxiety and depression. Relaxation techniques can promote a calmer, more positive outlook.
- **Increased Focus and Productivity**: Stress can cloud your thinking and hinder your ability to focus. Relaxation techniques can improve cognitive function and productivity.

- **Better Relationships**: Chronic stress can strain relationships. Cultivating inner peace can improve communication and strengthen your connections with others.

Your Stress Management Toolbox:

Here are some powerful techniques to incorporate into your daily routine for stress reduction and relaxation:

Mindfulness Meditation: Mindfulness involves focusing your attention on the present moment without judgment. It can help reduce stress, improve focus, and promote emotional well-being. There are numerous mindfulness apps and guided meditations available online to get you started.

Deep Breathing Exercises:

Deep breathing helps activate the relaxation response in your body, counteracting the fight-or-flight response triggered by stress. Try simple techniques like inhaling for a count of 4, holding for a count of 7, and exhaling slowly for a count of 8.

Progressive Muscle Relaxation: This technique involves progressively tensing and relaxing different muscle groups in your body. As you release the tension, you'll feel a sense of relaxation spreading throughout your body.

Yoga or Tai Chi: These mind-body practices combine gentle physical movements, breathing exercises, and meditation. They can be a powerful tool for stress reduction and overall well-being.

Spending Time in Nature: Immersing yourself in nature has proven benefits for reducing stress and promoting feelings of calm.

- Take a walk in the park,
- sit by a babbling brook, or
- simply spend time in your backyard appreciating the beauty of nature.

Engage in Activities You Enjoy: Make time for activities that bring you joy and a sense of relaxation. Whether it's reading, listening to music, spending time with loved ones, or pursuing a hobby, prioritize activities that help you unwind and de-stress.

Laughter is the Best Medicine: Laughter is a powerful stress reliever. Watch a funny movie, spend time with loved ones who make you laugh, or read a humorous book.

Finding What Works for You:

The key to effective stress management is to find techniques that resonate with you. Experiment with different methods and discover what helps you feel most relaxed and centered.

Building a Stress-Resilient Lifestyle:

Stress management isn't just about reacting to stress in the moment, but also about creating a lifestyle that promotes overall well-being. Here are some tips:

- **Set Realistic Goals:** Setting unrealistic goals can be a major source of stress. Set achievable goals and celebrate your progress along the way.
- **Practice Time Management**: Feeling overwhelmed by tasks can lead to stress. Learn effective time management techniques to

prioritize tasks and manage your workload efficiently.

- **Learn to Say No:** Don't be afraid to say no to requests that would overload you.
- **Maintain Strong Social Connections**: Having a strong support system is crucial for managing stress. Surround yourself with positive and supportive people who care about your well-being.
- **Seek Professional Help**: If you're struggling to manage stress on your own, don't hesitate to seek professional help from a therapist.

Chapter 14:

Building a Support System - The Power of Accountability and Encouragement on Your Weight Management Journey.

This chapter explores the importance of accountability and encouragement, and how surrounding yourself with positive influences can empower you to achieve your weight management goals and create lasting change.

Why You Need a Support System.

The road to lasting weight management can be challenging, filled with temptations and setbacks. A strong support system acts as a safety net, providing you with the accountability and encouragement you need to stay on track and reach your goals. Here's how:

Accountability: Sharing your goals with a trusted friend, family member, or support group creates a sense of accountability. Knowing someone believes in you and is invested in your success can be a powerful motivator to stay committed to your healthy lifestyle choices.

Motivation and Encouragement: Facing challenges and setbacks is inevitable. A support system can provide a steady stream of motivation and encouragement when you need it most. Positive reinforcement can help you overcome obstacles and persevere on your journey.

Shared Experiences: Connecting with others who are also on a weight management journey allows you to share experiences, swap tips, and offer each other support. Knowing you're not alone can be incredibly motivating and create a sense of familiarity.

Celebrating Successes: Reaching milestones, overcoming challenges, and achieving goals deserve to be celebrated! A support system allows you to share your victories and receive well-deserved recognition, boosting your confidence and motivation to keep moving forward.

Building Your Dream Team:

Here's how to cultivate a supportive network that empowers your weight management journey:

Identify Your "Cheerleaders": Look for individuals who are positive, supportive, and genuinely invested in your well-being. These are the people who will celebrate your successes, encourage you during setbacks, and hold you accountable for your choices.

Consider a Weight Loss Buddy: Finding a friend or family member who shares your goals can be a powerful motivator. Partner up for workouts, share recipes, or simply hold each other accountable for healthy habits.

Join a Support Group: Support groups provide a safe space to connect with others on a similar journey. You can share experiences, learn from each other, and find encouragement and motivation from a wider community. Online support groups can be a convenient option if in-person groups are not readily available.

Seek Professional Guidance: A registered dietitian, nutritionist, or certified personal trainer can provide valuable guidance, create a personalized plan, and offer support throughout your weight management journey.

Communication is Key:

Building a support system requires effective communication. Be open with your support network about your goals, challenges, and needs. Let them know how they can best support you, whether it's holding you accountable, providing encouragement, or simply being a listening ear.

The Strength of Positive Influence:

Surrounding yourself with positive and supportive people has a significant impact on your overall well-being. A strong support system can:

- **Boost Confidence**: Knowing you have people who believe in you can significantly enhance your confidence and self-esteem.
- **Reduce Stress**: A supportive network can help you manage stress more effectively, which is crucial for weight management success.

- **Improve Overall Health**: The positive energy and healthy habits of your support system can rub off on you, leading to a healthier lifestyle overall.

Remember: Building a support system is a two-way street. Offer encouragement and support to those in your network who are also working towards their health goals. Fostering a culture of mutual support creates a stronger and more impactful network for everyone involved.

Finally, building a strong support system isn't just about finding people to cheer you on. It's about creating a network of accountability, encouragement, and shared experiences. By surrounding yourself with positive influences, you empower yourself to achieve lasting change, embrace a healthier lifestyle, and reach your belly fat reduction goals, and ultimately, live a happier and healthier life.

Chapter 15:

Staying Motivated and Overcoming Plateaus - Reigniting Your Inner Flame on the Road to Success

Now, let's address a crucial aspect of any long-term journey: staying motivated and overcoming plateaus. This chapter equips you with effective strategies to reignite your inner flame, navigate inevitable setbacks, and maintain momentum as you strive for lasting weight management success.

The Inevitability of Plateaus:

Plateaus are a natural occurrence in any weight loss journey. They represent periods where the scale seems stuck, progress stalls, and motivation might dwindle. These plateaus, however, don't signify failure. They are simply signals to adjust your approach and reignite your commitment to your healthy lifestyle goals.

Why Motivation Wanes:

Understanding why motivation wanes can help you identify areas to address:

Monotony: Sticking to the same diet and exercise routine for an extended period can become monotonous, leading to boredom and a decreased desire to continue.

Setbacks: Everyone experiences setbacks. An unhealthy meal, a missed workout, or unexpected life events can derail your momentum and leave you feeling discouraged.

Loss of Focus: Life gets busy. Over time, the initial excitement of starting a new weight management program can fade, leading to a lack of focus on your goals.

Strategies to Reignite Your Motivation:

Here's your toolkit for staying motivated and overcoming plateaus:

- **Revisit Your Goals**: Take time to revisit your initial goals. Why did you embark on this journey? Reconnecting with your 'why' can reignite your passion and purpose.
- **Celebrate Non-Scale Victories**: Don't solely focus on the numbers on the scale. Celebrate non-scale victories like increased energy levels, improved strength, or better fitting clothes. Recognizing these positive changes keeps you motivated.
- **Mix Things Up:** ** Incorporate variety into your diet and exercise routine. Explore new healthy

recipes, try different workout styles, or join a fitness class. Novelty sparks excitement and keeps you engaged.

- **Set Short-Term Goals**: Break down your larger goals into smaller, achievable milestones. Accomplishing smaller goals provides a sense of accomplishment and keeps you motivated to reach your ultimate target.
- **Track Your Progress**: Keeping a food journal or workout log allows you to track your progress, identify areas for improvement, and celebrate your achievements.
- **Reward Yourself**: Celebrate milestones with non-food rewards like a massage, a new workout outfit, or a fun activity. Rewarding yourself reinforces positive habits and keeps you motivated.
- **Find Inspiration**:** Surround yourself with positive influences.

Seek out inspirational stories, read success blogs, or follow motivational figures on social media.

- **Don't Be Afraid to Seek Help**: If motivation remains elusive, reach out to your support network, a registered dietitian, or a therapist. Talking to someone can help you identify challenges and develop strategies to overcome them.

Embracing Setbacks as Stepping Stones:

Setbacks are inevitable. The key is to view them as temporary roadblocks and not permanent derailments. Here's how to bounce back from setbacks:

Acknowledge the Setback: Don't beat yourself up. Recognize the setback, learn from it, and move forward.

Get Back on Track Quickly: Don't let one unhealthy meal turn into a week of indulgence. Get back on track with your next meal or workout.

Focus on Progress, Not Perfection: Aim for progress, not perfection. There will be bumps along the road, but consistent effort leads to success.

Developing   Long-Term Sustainability:
Remember, weight management isn't about a quick fix; it's about creating a sustainable and healthy lifestyle. Here are some tips:

Focus on Healthy Habits:** Focus on building healthy habits that you can maintain for the long term. Don't view this as a temporary diet, but rather a lifestyle change.
Make Gradual Changes: Making drastic changes is difficult to sustain.

Introduce healthy changes gradually to allow your body and mind to adapt.

Find Activities You Enjoy: Choose dietary choices and exercise routines that you genuinely enjoy. This increases the likelihood of sticking with them in the long term.

Practice Self-Compassion: Be kind to yourself. There will be slip-ups. The key is to learn, adjust, and keep moving forward.

Conclusion: Reigniting Your Journey to a Healthier You

We've reached the culmination of your comprehensive guide to fat reduction after 40. Throughout this journey, you've delved into the science, explored practical strategies, and built a foundation for lasting success. Now, let's solidify your learnings with a recap of key takeaways, establish a long-term vision for health and well-being, and explore resources to propel you forward on your path.

Recap of Key Strategies:

This guide has equipped you with a powerful toolkit for fat reduction and overall health improvement. Here's a quick recap of the essential strategies we've explored:

Understanding Hormonal Changes: You've learned how hormonal shifts, particularly after the age of 40, can influence weight management.

Crafting a Balanced Diet: We've explored the importance of macronutrients – protein, carbohydrates, and healthy fats – and mindful eating practices for sustainable weight management.

Incorporating Enjoyable Exercise: You've discovered the importance of finding exercise routines you love, promoting consistency and boosting motivation.

Prioritizing Quality Sleep: You've learned how sleep deprivation disrupts hormones, metabolism, and appetite control, highlighting the importance of prioritizing restful sleep.

Managing Stress and Finding Calm: We've discussed the negative impact of stress on weight management and explored effective techniques for stress reduction and relaxation.

Building a Support System: You've learned the value of a supportive network for accountability, encouragement, and shared experiences.

Staying Motivated and Overcoming Plateaus: We've equipped you with strategies to navigate inevitable plateaus, reignite motivation, and maintain focus on your goals.

Long-Term Vision for Health and Well-being:

Maintaining a healthy weight after 40 is just one aspect of a broader journey towards lifelong health and well-being. By incorporating the strategies outlined in this guide, you'll experience benefits that extend beyond fat loss:

Increased Energy Levels: Healthy eating, quality sleep, and regular exercise all contribute to increased energy levels throughout the day.

Improved Mood: Prioritizing your health can lead to a more positive outlook and improved emotional well-being.

Reduced Risk of Chronic Diseases: A healthy lifestyle lowers your risk of developing chronic conditions like heart disease, diabetes, and certain cancers.

Enhanced Confidence: As you progress on your journey, you'll gain confidence in your ability to make healthy choices and achieve your goals.

Overall Sense of Well-being: By prioritizing your physical and mental health, you'll cultivate a sense of well-being that impacts all aspects of your life.

Embrace the Ongoing Journey:

Remember, weight management and overall health improvement are lifelong journeys. Embrace the ongoing process, celebrate your victories, learn from setbacks, and maintain your commitment to a healthy lifestyle.

Taking Action:

Here are some concrete steps you can take to move forward:

Create a personalized action plan: Review the strategies outlined in this guide and choose those that resonate most with you. Develop a personalized action plan to incorporate these strategies into your daily routine.

Set realistic and achievable goals: Break down your long-term goals into smaller, manageable steps. Celebrate achieving these milestones to stay motivated on your journey.

Share your goals with your support system: Let your support network know about your goals and how they can best support you. Their encouragement can be a powerful motivator.

Be patient and persistent: Remember, lasting change takes time and commitment. Be patient with yourself and celebrate your progress, big or small.

Lastly, you now possess the knowledge and tools to embark on a transformative journey towards a healthier and happier you. Embrace the process, celebrate your victories, and never lose sight of

Bonus Section:

Sample Meal Plans and Workout Routines Tailored for Different Needs and Preferences.

This bonus section provides sample meal plans and workout routines designed to cater to various dietary needs and exercise preferences. Remember, these are just examples, and you should always personalize your plan based on your specific goals, calorie needs, and any allergies or dietary restrictions. It's recommended to consult a registered dietitian or certified personal trainer for a plan tailored to your unique situation.

Sample Meal Plans:

1. Balanced Diet (1500 Calories):

Breakfast (400 calories): Greek yogurt with berries and granola, whole-wheat toast with avocado and eggs.

Lunch (500 calories): Grilled chicken salad with mixed greens, quinoa, and vegetables with a light vinaigrette dressing.

Dinner (600 calories): Salmon with roasted vegetables and brown rice.

2. Vegetarian Option (1800 Calories):

Breakfast (450 calories): Whole-wheat pancakes with fruit and nuts, tofu scramble with vegetables.

Lunch (550 calories): Lentil soup with whole-grain bread, veggie burger on a whole-wheat bun with roasted sweet potato fries.

Dinner (800 calories): Vegetarian chili with brown rice and avocado, side salad with balsamic vinaigrette.

3. High-Protein Option (2000 Calories):

Breakfast (500 calories): Eggs with spinach and whole-wheat toast, protein smoothie with berries and Greek yogurt.
Lunch (600 calories): Grilled chicken breast with brown rice and steamed broccoli, side salad with olive oil and vinegar.
Dinner (900 calories): Baked salmon with roasted asparagus and quinoa, protein salad with grilled chicken, vegetables, and quinoa.

Sample Workout Routines:

1. Beginner Cardio and Strength Training (30 Minutes):

- 15 minutes brisk walking or light jogging,

- Bodyweight exercises circuit (3 sets of 10-12 repetitions): squats, lunges, push-ups (modified if needed), rows, sit-ups (modified if needed).

2. HIIT (High-Intensity Interval Training) for Experienced Individuals (20 Minutes):

- **Warm-up**: 5 minutes of light cardio (e.g., jogging, jumping jacks)
- Alternate between high-intensity exercises (e.g., sprinting, burpees, jumping squats) for 30 seconds each and rest periods of 30 seconds.
- Cool-down: 5 minutes of light stretching

3. Strength Training Focus (45 Minutes):

- Major muscle groups (legs, back, chest, shoulders, core) with compound exercises (e.g., squats, deadlifts, bench press, rows) using weights for 3 sets of 8-12 repetitions each.
- Light cardio for cool-down (10-15 minutes).

Additional Tips:

- Always consult your doctor before starting a new exercise program.
- Listen to your body and take rest days when needed.
- Gradually increase intensity and duration of workouts as you get fitter.
- Explore different exercise styles like yoga, Pilates, or swimming to find activities you enjoy.
- Make it a habit to stay active throughout the day with activities like taking the stairs or going for a walk during breaks.

Remember, consistency is key! By incorporating these strategies into your routine and adapting them to your preferences, you'll be well on your way to achieving your belly fat reduction goals and creating a healthier, happier you.